Ancient Method To Dissolve Kidney Stones

By: Jack Kevin

Disclaimer

graphics contained in this Book for any purpose. Any use of this information is at your own risk.

This Book contains information that is intended to help the readers be better informed of health care. Always consult your doctor for individual needs.

The Book is not intended to be a substitute for the medical advice of licensed physician. The reader should consult with their doctor in any matters relating to his/her health.

By using anything found in this eBook and using it, it is at your own risk, you take full responsibility for your actions, if you don't agree or don't want to take your own risk than is suggest you overlook this report.

Table of contents

Introduction

Hi Dear Readers am Jack Kevin author of "Ancient Method To Dissolve Kidney Stones". Thanks for Buying this Book. This Book provide information for treating kidney stone and eliminating them from the body forever and it will never let them happen to form again in future. The information in this Book is Collected from my own personal research and specially the Indian Veda called Ayurveda and all the information in this Book is ancient and you will never get this information elsewhere because the all information was in Hindi language and ancient Sanskrit for that I have translated all the information to English. This Book cover information regarding kidney stone, there types, causes, food to avoid, Treatment for kidney stone, Operations regarding kidney stones, and ancient natural remedies and method to dissolve the kidney stone so that you don't have to go for operation and you can easily eliminate kidney stone at home.

What are kidney stones?

Kidney stones also called renal calculi, are crystals solid products. Kidney stones develops in your both kidneys at any time. However, they can be also produced or developed anywhere in your urinary tract, which consists of these parts:

- kidneys
- ureters
- bladder
- urethra

Kidney stones are one of the most painful medical conditions. The causes of kidney stones vary according to the Different type of stone.

Kidney stones takes place because of build-up of dissolved minerals on the inner lining of the kidneys.

They commonly consist of calcium oxalate but may be composed of several other compounds.

Kidney stones can grow to the size of a golf ball while maintaining a sharp, crystalline structure.

The stones may be small and pass unnoticed through the urinary tract, but they can also cause extreme pain as they leave the body.

Causes

Kidney stones can vary in size. Some have been known to grow as large as golf balls size.

The Major cause of kidney stones is a lack of water in the body.

Stones are most commonly found in individuals who drink less than the recommended eight to ten glasses of water a day.

When there is not enough water to dilute the uric acid, a component of urine, the urine becomes more acidic. An excessively acidic environment in urine can lead to the formation of kidney stones. Medical conditions such as Crohn's disease, urinary tract infections, renal tubular acidosis, hyperparathyroidism, medullary sponge kidney, and Dent's disease increase the risk of kidney stones.

Types of kidney stones

Not all types kidney stones are made up of the same crystals. The different types of kidney stones include:

Calcium

Calcium stones are the most commonly found in major number. They're mostly made of calcium oxalate (though they can consist of calcium phosphate or maleate). Eating fewer oxalate-rich foods can reduce your risk of developing this type of stone. High-oxalate foods include:

- potato chips
- peanuts
- chocolate
- beets
- spinach

However, even though some kidney stones are made of calcium, getting enough calcium in your diet can prevent stones from forming.

Uric acid

This type of kidney stone is more common in men than in women. They can occur in people with gout or those going through chemotherapy. This type of stone develops when urine is too acidic. A diet rich in purines can increase urine's acidic level. Purine is a colorless substance in animal proteins, such as fish, shellfish, and meats.

Struvite

This type of stone is found mostly in women with urinary tract infections (UTIs). These stones can be large and cause urinary obstruction. They result from a kidney infection. Treating an underlying infection can prevent the development of struvite stones.

Cystine

Cystine stones are rare. They occur in both men and women who have the genetic disorder cystinuria. With this type of stone, cystine — an acid that occurs naturally in the body — leaks from the kidneys into the urine.

Risk factors for kidney stones

The greatest risk factor for kidney stones is making less than one liter of urine per day. This is why kidney stones are common in premature infants who have kidney problems. However, kidney stones are most likely to occur in people between the ages of 20 and 50.

Different factors can increase your risk of developing a stone. Typically, Caucasians are more likely to have kidney stones than those of African descent.

More men than women develop kidney stones, according to the National Institute of Diabetes and Digestive and Kidney Diseases (NIDDK).

A history of kidney stones can increase your risk. So does a family history of kidney stones.

Certain medications can increase the risk of developing kidney stones. Scientists found that topiramate , a drug commonly prescribed to treat seizures and migraine headaches, can increase the likelihood of kidney stones developing.

Additionally, it is possible that long-term use of vitamin D and calcium supplements cause high calcium levels, which can contribute to kidney stones.

Additional risk factors for kidney stones include diets that are high in protein and sodium but low in calcium, a sedentary lifestyle, obesity, high blood pressure, and conditions that affect how calcium is absorbed in the body such as gastric bypass surgery, inflammatory bowel disease, and chronic diarrhea.

Other risk factors include:

- dehydration
- obesity
- a diet with high levels of protein, salt, or glucose
- hyperparathyroid condition

- gastric bypass surgery
- inflammatory bowel diseases that increase calcium absorption
- taking medications such as diuretics, antiseizure drugs, and calcium-based antacids

Recognizing the symptoms and signs of a kidney stone

Kidney stones are known to cause severe pain. Symptoms of kidney stones may not occur until the stone begins to move down the ureters. This severe pain is called renal colic. You may have pain on one side of your back or abdomen.

In men, pain may radiate to the groin area. The pain of renal colic comes and goes, but can be intense. People with renal colic tend to be restless.

Other symptoms of kidney stones can include:

- blood in the urine (red, pink, or brown urine)
- vomiting
- nausea
- discolored or foul-smelling urine

- chills
- fever
- frequent need to urinate
- urinating small amounts of urine
- severe pain in the groin and/or side
- blood in urine
- vomiting and nausea
- white blood cells or pus in the urine
- reduced amount of urine excreted
- burning sensation during urination
- persistent urge to urinate
- fever and chills if there is an infection

In the case of a small kidney stone, you may not have any pain or symptoms as the stone passes through your urinary tract.

Testing for and diagnosing kidney stones

Diagnosis of kidney stones requires a complete health history assessment and a physical exam. Other tests include:

- blood tests for calcium, phosphorus, uric acid, and electrolytes
- blood urea nitrogen (BUN) and creatinine to assess kidney functioning
- urinalysis to check for crystals, bacteria, blood, and white cells
- examination of passed stones to determine their type

The following tests can rule out obstruction:

- abdominal X-rays
- intravenous pyelogram (IVP)
- retrograde pyelogram
- ultrasound of the kidney (the preferred study)

- MRI scan of the abdomen and kidneys
- abdominal CT scan

The contrast dye used in the CT scan and the IVP can affect kidney function. However, in people with normal kidney function, this isn't a concern.

There are some medications that can increase the potential for kidney damage in conjunction with the dye. Make sure your radiologist knows about any medications you're taking.

How kidney stones are treated

Treatment is tailored according to the type of stone. Urine can be strained and stones collected for evaluation.

Drinking six to eight glasses of water a day increases urine flow. People who are dehydrated or have severe nausea and vomiting may need intravenous fluids.

Other treatment options include:

Medication

Pain relief may require narcotic medications. The presence of infection requires treatment with antibiotics. Other medications include:

- allopurinol (Zyloprim) for uric acid stones
- diuretics
- sodium bicarbonate or sodium citrate
- phosphorus solutions
- ibuprofen (Advil)

- acetaminophen (Tylenol)
- naproxen sodium (Aleve)

Lithotripsy

Extracorporeal shock wave lithotripsy uses sound waves to break up large stones so they can more easily pass down the ureters into your bladder. This procedure can be uncomfortable and may require light anesthesia. It can cause bruising on the abdomen and back and bleeding around the kidney and nearby organs.

Tunnel surgery (percutaneous nephrolithotomy)

Stones are removed through a small incision in your back. This procedure and may be needed when:

- the stone causes obstruction and infection or is damaging the kidneys
- the stone has grown too large to pass
- pain can't be controlled

Ureteroscopy

When a stone is stuck in the ureter or bladder, your doctor may use an instrument called a ureteroscope to remove it. A small wire with a camera attached is inserted into the urethra and passed into the bladder. The doctor then uses a small cage to snag the stone and remove it. The stone is then sent to the laboratory for analysis.

Kidney stone prevention

Proper hydration is a key preventive measure. We recommends drinking enough water to pass about 2.6 quarts of urine each day. Increasing the amount of urine you pass helps flush the kidneys.

You can substitute ginger ale, lemon-lime soda, and fruit juice for water to help you increase your fluid intake. If the stones are related to low citrate levels, citrate juices could help prevent the formation of stones.

Eating oxalate-rich foods in moderation and reducing your intake of salt and animal proteins can also lower your risk of kidney stones.

Your doctor may prescribe medications to help prevent the formation of calcium and uric acid stones. If you've had a kidney stone or you're at risk for a kidney stone, speak with your doctor and discuss the best methods of prevention.

How to prevent kidney stones naturally

Making small adjustments to your current diet and nutrition plan may go a long way toward preventing kidney stones.

1. Stay hydrated

Drinking more water is the best way to prevent kidney stones. If you don't drink enough, your urine output will be low. Low urine output means your urine is more concentrated and less likely to dissolve urine salts that cause stones.

Lemonade and orange juice are also good options. They both contain citrate, which may prevent stones from forming.

Try to drink around eight glasses of fluids daily, or enough to pass two liters of urine. If you exercise or sweat a lot, or if you have a history of cystine stones, you'll need additional fluids.

You can tell whether you're hydrated by looking at the color of your urine — it should be clear or pale yellow. If it's dark, you need to drink more.

2. Eat more calcium-rich foods

The most common type of kidney stone is the calcium oxalate stone, leading many people to believe they should avoid eating calcium. The opposite is true. Low-calcium diets may increase your kidney stone risk and your risk of osteoporosis.

Calcium supplements, however, may increase your risk of stones. Taking calcium supplements with a meal may help reduce that risk.

Low-fat milk, low-fat cheese, and low-fat yogurt are all good calcium-rich food options.

3. Eat less sodium

A high-salt diet increases your risk of calcium kidney stones. According to the Urology Care Foundation, too much salt in the urine prevents calcium from being reabsorbed from the urine to the blood. This causes high urine calcium, which may lead to kidney stones.

Eating less salt helps keep urine calcium levels lower. The lower the urine calcium, the lower the risk of developing kidney stones.

To reduce your sodium intake, read food labels carefully.

Foods notorious for being high in sodium include:

- processed foods, such as chips and crackers
- canned soups
- canned vegetables
- lunch meat
- condiments

- foods that contain monosodium glutamate
- foods that contain sodium nitrate
- foods that contain sodium bicarbonate (baking soda)

To flavor foods without using salt, try fresh herbs or a salt-free, herbal seasoning blend.

4. Eat fewer oxalate-rich foods

Some kidney stones are made of oxalate, a natural compound found in foods that binds with calcium in the urine to form kidney stones. Limiting oxalate-rich foods may help prevent the stones from forming.

Foods high in oxalates are:

- spinach
- chocolate
- sweet potatoes
- coffee
- beets
- peanuts
- rhubarb
- soy products
- wheat bran

Oxalate and calcium bind together in the digestive tract before reaching the kidneys, so it's harder for stones to form if you eat high-oxalate foods and calcium-rich foods at the same time.

5. Eat less animal protein

Foods high in animal protein are acidic and may increase urine acid. High urine acid may cause both uric acid and calcium oxalate kidney stones.

You should try to limit or avoid:

- beef
- poultry
- fish
- pork

6. Avoid vitamin C supplements

Vitamin C (ascorbic acid) supplementation may cause kidney stones, especially in men.

According to one 2013 study, men who took high doses of vitamin C supplements doubled their risk of forming a kidney stone.

Researchers don't believe vitamin C from food carries the same risk.

7. Explore herbal remedies

Chanca Piedra, also known as the "stone breaker," is a popular herbal folk remedy for kidney stones. The herb is thought to help prevent calcium-oxalate stones from forming. It's also believed to reduce the size of existing stones.

Use herbal remedies with caution. They're not well-regulated or well-researched for the prevention or treatment of kidney stones.

Ancient Remedies to dissolve the kidney stone permanently

1. Hazrul yahud bhasma

(Calcium silicate or Lime Silicate)

Hazrul yahud bhasma is a Ayurvedic-induced medicine that is used in kidney stones, urine and nervous system which is also known as Sange yahud Bhasma, Ber patthar bhasma, Bharashma Bhasma, Hazrul yahud Bhasma or Calclined Lime Silicate. These stones are fossil stones. The main structure of these stones is Lime Silicates.

Medical properties

The following are the main health and therapeutic properties of Hajarul yahud bhasma.

1. Diuretic
2. Stone dusters (Dissolves stones in the kidneys or bladder)
3. Kandoorodi (the pestilence
4. Painkiller (effective in renal)

Kidney stones and renal duct

Hazrul yahud, has diuretic functions in the body, helps in smelting and pushing the kidney stones during urine. The most important thing is that it also has painkillers, which reduces renal failure within the first 2 to 3 doses.

Urine Crystal (urine leaving crystal)

Crystalline is a condition in which crystals are found in urine. This is due to the side effects of stones in urine or some medicines. The cause of crystalluria is due to medicines like penicillin and sulfomamide. In this situation, Hazrul yahud bhasma provides

Chandraprabha Vati benefits with Jadam Bhasam. One month course of these remedies eliminates crystalline. If crystallization of crystalline occurs repeatedly, then these remedies should be done for a minimum of three months. In addition, the use of Chandnasav in treatment also gives benefit in the form of co-drug.

Quantity and consumption method (dosage)
The amount of dose of Hazrul yahud bhasma varies according to the condition of the patient's health and age. Normal dose ranges from 250 mg to 500 mg twice a day. The maximum amount of Hazrul yahud Bhasma supplements should not be more than 2 grams per day.

Dosage
Minimum effective dose of 125 mg (in children) 250 mg (in adults) *
Medium dose (adult) 250 mg to 500 mg *
Medium dose (baby) 125 mg to 250 mg *

Maximum potential dose 2000 mg **
* Twice a day ** total daily dose divided amounts

Consumption method

2 times - morning and evening
With lukewarm water.

Treatment period

For at least 3 months.

Caution and Side Effects

There is no authentic information about the side effects of Hazrul yahud bhasma and its use in pregnancy and breastfeeding. Avoid using Hazrul yahud Bhasma in pregnancy and stay safe.

2. Gokshura(Tribulus terrestris)

Gokshura is also known as Tribulus terrestris which is widely distributed in the world and only grows in dry climate where only a few plants can survive. It is considered an invasive species in North America. Gokshura is an herbaceous taprooted perennial plant which grows in summer in colder climates. This plant can also thrive in poor soil conditions and desert climates. It can also be found in Australia, Africa, Southern Asia and Southern Europe. The stem of this plant grows around 10 centimetres in diameter and usually forms flat patches. The stem branch is usually hairy and the leaves are pinnately compound. The leaflets are around 3 mm long.

Gokshura is very beneficial in curing urinary diseases and kidney stones. Regular consumption of Gokshura can easily relieve a person from bladder problems and diuretic ailments. The diuretic activity of Gokshura is well utilized through a lot of formulations. It has a cleansing effect on the urinary bladder. This is because Gokshura is filled with lithotryptic activity which helps in regulating the functioning of the urinary system.

According to Ayurveda, the quantity of potassium and nitrate in Gokshura is very high and it has diuretic properties. It breaks the kidney stones into small pieces and helps them to get out of the urinary tract and also increases the amount of uric acid. In this regard, regular consumption of Gokshura is beneficial in kidney stones and other related diseases of the kidneys.

How much and how much quantity should be consumed?

Gokhru or Gokshura is available in three different forms: Gokshura powders, Gokhshura Kwath, Gokshur Tablet.

-Gokshura powder: half a teaspoon with milk twice a day.

-Gokshura Kawth: After mixing equal quantity of water in 15-30 ml gokshura kawth, after eating twice a day, take it.

Gokshura tablet: Take one to two capsules daily after feeding with milk twice a day.

Is it beneficial to use Gokshrua with milk?

Yes, by consuming Gokshrua with milk, its benefits increases.

What are the Gokshura side effects

If you consume Gokshura for a limited period, then there is no side effect. Consumption of excess amounts of Gokshura for a long time can cause problems in stomach, vomiting, nausea, diarrhea and sleep problems.

3. Daikon Juice

White Radish belongs to the family of root vegetables. It tastes acrid, sour, and pungent and has peppery flavor.
Radish is available in four varieties Red, White, Black and yellow.
It was cultivated in Europe initially. Also widely cultivated in Asia.

Fresh Radish juice of 50 to 100 grams mixed with little sugar and taken early in the morning will give relief from kidney pains in 3 to 4 days.

If taken for 3 to 4 weeks it gradually dissolves stones in kidneys and urinary tract.

Side Effects and Precautions of Daikon White Radish

Radish should not be taken along with fish or black gram. Milk should not be taken soon after taking radish.

4. Yavakshara

(Carbonate of Potash or Potassium Carbonate)

Yavakshara is an Ayurvedic medicine, used in dissolving kidney stones treating urinary diseases, abdominal pain, bloating, etc . Yava kshar is potassium carbonate K_2CO_3 a white salt. It is also used as ingredient in many medicines. Yava kshara alkali preparation made with whole plant of barley (botanical name – Hordeum vulgare). Here barley – whole plant is dried, burnt in open air, ash is added with water, left over night. Sedimented portion is discarded and decanted clear liquid is filtered many times.

After getting a clear liquid, it is heated and the solid powder which is leftover at the bottom of the vessel is called as Yavakshara.

Synonyms:

Yav Ksar, Jav Kshar, Jav Ksar, Yavaksaram, Yavaja, Yavashukaja

Yavahva, Yavya, Yavagraja

Pakya, Pakya Kshara

YavaKshara (an alkali preparation from the plant barley) is useful in

Hrudroga – heart diseases,

Pandu – anemia,

Grahani – malabsoprtion syndrome (IBS)

Pleeha – enlargement of spleen,

Anaha – bloating, constipation,

Galagraha – obstruction in throat,

Kasa – coughing and

Kaphaja Ashmari – piles of Slaismika variety.

Yava Kshara Dosage:

125 mg – 500 mg used in various combination, for oral intake and also for external application.

Yavakshara side effects:

It is best to avoid in high Pitta conditions, bleeding disorders, as it is hot, strong and piercing in nature.

Since it is a Kshara, it is best avoided in men seeking treatment for infertility, as it may affect the quality and quantity of sperm production.

In higher doses, it may cause burning sensation.

It is not ideal to use this medicine in people with excessive tiredness, emaciation and who are underweight.

Yava kshara ingredients:

Yava – Barley – Hordeum vulgare

How to make Yava Kshar?

Whole plant of Barley (Hordeum vulgare) are collected, cleaned well, dried completely in sunlight.

It is taken in a big iron pan and burnt completely in open air.

After it cools down on its own, the ash is collected and mixed with 4 times of water (6 times of water according to other reference) then mixed well, filtered with cloth, into an Iron vessel.

These contents are kept for one night as it is.

Next day morning the clear supernatent part of water is filtered with a cloth into another vessel.

This process of filtering is repeated for 3 – 4 times.

Then this water is heated over mild fire, till the water content gets totally evaporated.

White colored Yava Kshar is produced. It is stored in an air tight glass contained. Yava kshar is potassium carbonate K2CO3 a white salt.

If you can't produce Yava kshar at home then you can buy potassium carbonate from Medical shop.

5. Kalmi Shora

(Nitrate of Potash or Potassium Nitrate)

Kalmi Shora is known as Salt Peter in English and its chemical name is called KNO_3. Its look like ordinary salt, used in many recipes. It can dissolve kidney stones easily without going for surgery. Regular consumption of kalmi shora can dissolve kidney stone naturally upto 20 mm. you can buy potassium nitrate from medical shop.

Take 1-2 gm twice daily on empty stomach with water.

6. Shwet parpati

Shwet Parpati is used for Urinary tract infections, Painful urination and other conditions.

Shwet Parpati improves the patient's condition by performing the following functions:

- Increasing urine output and blood flow in kidneys.

Before using Shwet Parpati, inform your doctor about your current list of medications, over the counter products (e.g. vitamins, herbal supplements, etc.), allergies, pre-existing diseases, and current health conditions (e.g. pregnancy, upcoming surgery, etc.). Some health conditions may make you more susceptible to the side-effects of the drug. Take as directed by your doctor or follow the direction printed on the product insert. Dosage is based on your condition. Tell your doctor if your condition persists or worsens. Important counseling points are listed below.

- Bleeding disorders

Hypersensitivity to Shwet Parpati is a contraindication. In addition, Shwet Parpati should not be used if you have the following conditions:

- Children
- Lactating mothers
- Pregnant

Dosage: 1 to 4 grams per day

How to make shwet parpati:

Ingredients:

1. Alum (KAI(SO4)2.12H2O) = 50 grams

2. Potassium Nitrate (KNO3) = 400 grams

3. Ammonia (NH4CL) = 25 grams

Take all the ingredients together in a clay vessel and put it on high flame stir well till it become liquid then take the molten liquid and put it on banana tree leaf and after that put another banana leaf to cover the molten liquid which is on banana leaf and instantly press the liquid between

two banana leaf with something like plate
etc to make it solidify in between two
leafs and then allow to cool your shwet
parpati is ready to use.

Secret ancient formulation to remove kidney stone

If the Kidney stone is equal to the chicken egg then this formulation will remove that.

Ingredients: Hazrul yahud bhasma 50 gram, Kalami Shora 100 grams, Daikon juice 3 kg

.

Collect all these medicines. Divide the kalmi shora into two parts, 50-50 grams, and divide the Daikon juice into 6 parts (500 - 500 gm.). Now before all, put 50 grams of kalmi shora in a clay vessel, Add half a kilo Daikon juice on it. Add 50 grams of kalmi shora to it again.

Put the ingredients in clay utensil put it on flame. Stop the flame when the solution is remained only 500 grams. Put Daikon juice and again cook it in on flame. This is to be done by 6 times which is to pour Daikon juice. After giving full flame the Formulation is ready.

Take the above-mentioned medication with 2 grains, Yavakshara 2 grains, mooli kshara 2 grains, and feed them three times a day with water. The kidney stones are easily removed with this formulation

1 grain is 0.06 grams. Thus, the above mentioned Formulation is to take 2 gran = 0.12 gram three, that is, together with all three 0.36 grams. Take it more than 1 gram.

Method of making yavakshar An Ayurvdic Medicine

Yavakshara or barley is light brown in color. Due to boiling the ash in water, it becomes a very good medicine for kidney patients.

Yavakshar can be made of two types.

First method of making yavakshara

Take out half-baked barley plants and cut them into pieces. Burn it out to make ashes. Mix the water in the ash thoroughly. Leave it for 6-7 hours. Keep stirring well between the middle beach. Finally when the water cools down, then remove the straws from the top and drain the water. Gradually lower the remaining white colored liquid on low flame slowly. When it gets thick enough, dry it. This is what is called a little powdered yavakshara.

Second method of making yavakshara

In this method Barley is used instead of Barley Plant. Burn the barley first and make its ashes. Mix the water in the ash thoroughly. Keep it for 10-15 minutes. Shake again and keep it for 10-15 minutes. Do it four to five times. Then drain the water and throw it. Gradually lower the remaining white colored liquid on low flame slowly. When it gets thick enough, dry it. This is what is called a little powdered yavakshara.

Method of preparation of Mooli kshar

To make Mooli kshar, cut the radish and dry
them in the shade. Then burn them and
make them ashes. Add 8 times water to this
ash and keep it for 6-7 hours. Keep shaking
in between. After this, drain the top.
Gradually cook this diluted fluid slowly on a
low flame. The bottom of which remains a
bit residual, the same radish is alkali. Keep it
dry. It is used for many diseases.

If you have Kidney stones, take Mooli kshar
in the morning or take a cup of radish juice
in the morning and take an empty stomach
in the morning. There will also be less
chance of making stones again

Staying hydrated is key

Drinking plenty of fluids is a vital part of
passing kidney stones and preventing new
stones from forming. Not only does the

liquid flush out toxins, it helps move stones and grit through your urinary tract.

Although water alone may be enough to do the trick, adding certain ingredients can be beneficial. Be sure to drink one 8-ounce glass of water immediately after drinking any flavored remedy. This can help move the ingredients through your system.

Talk to your doctor before getting started with any of the home remedies listed below. They can assess whether home treatment is right for you or if it could lead to additional complications.

If you're pregnant or breastfeeding, avoid using any remedies. Your doctor can determine whether a juice may cause side effects for you or your baby.

When passing a stone, upping your water intake can help speed up the process. Strive for 12 glasses of water per day instead of the usual 8.

Once the stone passes, you should continue to drink 8 to 12 glasses of water each day.

Dehydration is one of the main risk factors for kidney stones, and the last thing you want is for more to form.

Pay attention to the color of your urine. It should be a very light, pale yellow. Dark yellow urine is a sign of dehydration.

Conclusion

Thank you for making it through to the end of "Ancient Method to Dissolve Kidney Stones", I hope it was informative and was able to provide you with all remedies you need to get rid of kidney stones. The next step is to start trying some of these ancient remedies for your kidney stone disease. Start with one or two and see what works best to dissolve kidney stone fast. Make sure that you follow recommended doses, Indication and warning; otherwise, you may not get any relief. It's also a good idea to talk to your doctor first. Finally, if you found this eBook useful in any way, a review on amazon is always appreciated. This book is to help people eliminate kidney stone and if you can not make the remedies given in this Book by yourself then you can buy them from chemical shop, medical shop or herbs shop which has imported herbs from different countries, and if you can not find these herbs from your near area then you can buy them online

For more information check our

Facebook page:
www.facebook.com/Health.fitness.blogg

Twitter page:

www.twitter.com/Hbloggg

Instagram:
www.instagram.com/Health.fitness.bloggg

Website:

 www.healthfitnessblogg.com